WHOLESOME HABITS

Shaping Routines Grounded in Values

By

Dr. Andreas Svoboda

Table of Content

INTRODUCTION

Hello there, beautiful being!

Try to picture a life where your routines are not mechanically accomplished items on a list but genuine expressions of your deepest convictions. A lovely setting in which regular activities become loving affirmations that reassure you, "Hey, I care about you." What do you think?

Let's take baby steps in this together. Developing healthy routines focuses on something other than making drastic changes. Nah-uh! It's gently shedding light on the minute, seemingly inconsequential decisions that subtly but significantly shape your daily existence. What's the deal with your daily cup of joe? That's a blank slate just begging to be painted with goodness.

Picture yourself switching from a quick espresso shot to a relaxing coffee routine. Envision yourself soaking in the morning sun as you leisurely stir your coffee and give yourself permission to just be. You're doing more than just making coffee; in fact, you create an oasis of calm with each cup.

To begin this journey, you must have a heart-to-heart with your ideals. What moves you deeply? Is it genuineness, friendliness, or willingness to take risks? Your good behaviors constantly prod you to be more authentic.

Let's have some fun with this: if spreading goodwill makes you feel good, try developing a daily routine that includes a small act of kindness. It could be as simple as sending a friend a heartfelt text message or as big as giving a total stranger your best grin. Straightforward, but oh, so effective!

Think of your routine actions as musical notes that move over the score of your life. What a beautiful symphony you compose when each note (habit) harmonizes with the melody (values)! The rhythmic beauty of your daily life will be woven with the pure habits you develop, my buddy.
Feeling adventurous? Awesome! But keep in mind that you're in no hurry. Maintaining healthy routines is not about being a perfectionist or following a list of "shoulds." They're gentle encouragement to follow your heart and live a life that makes your soul happy.

- **Identify:** Get comfortable in a secluded area and ask yourself softly, "What values nestle close to my heart?"

- **Imagine:** Envision a day where these principles effortlessly weave into all your activities. What do you think? How do you feel?

- **Integrate:** Incorporate them into your life by creating happy, small daily rituals that remind you of your values. Keep in mind that what really matters are small acts of kindness toward oneself.

Introducing Wholesome Habits

Healthy routines are like the countless twinkling lights that softly illuminate the night sky. They're not very big, but their light shines so brightly that it brightens the entire cosmos.

Developing and maintaining a positive routine requires more than just more work. It's a deliberate, thoughtful action that subtly advances you toward a life that chimes with your true self and core ideals. It's the tea you drink every day but with a little more mindfulness and happiness added in.

Picture your good routine as a warm breeze stroking your face and whispering true warmth and affection in your ear.

If kindness warms your soul, it could be a good practice to send a handwritten note of gratitude to the person who brightened your day. For you, self-care can involve allowing yourself to take a moment to pause and breathe deeply amid the chaos of the day.

No one has the right to coerce you into adopting healthy routines. Like pliable clay, they need to be worked carefully and painstakingly into their final form.

Get in touch with your feelings; tune in. Find out what it wants by listening to its heart's quiet, low rumbles. Think about small things you can do daily that will bring you happiness. Wholeheartedly embrace your healthy routine and allow it to shape your life rather than restrict it.

Use this mirror as a daily self-check. Your actions and ideals should be dancing together in harmony and beauty, so let your habits represent who you really are.

Envision your day being knit together with these lovely, thoughtful acts that mirror your deepest convictions and surround your life with soft, loving compassion. Isn't it stunning?

The Pertinence of Values in Habit Formation

Isn't it amazing that at the core of our daily actions beats intention and significance? Let's find a quiet spot and have a hearty discussion on something as simple as the importance of values in shaping healthy routines.

Just for a moment, pretend you're lost in a mysterious wilderness. Your morals? They are your map, leading the way through the lush vegetation so that each step you take harmonizes with your core values.

The term "values" refers to more than just ideas. They provide a cushioned but stable base while you move to the beat of life. Your principles, whether kindness, authenticity, or adventure, will determine how you move through this wonderful, unpredictable dance of life.

Visualize the fine threads of your values as the foundation upon which your daily actions are built. When a routine is tied to a principle, it stops feeling like a burden. Instead, it seems to flow easily and naturally from you.

Having a habit driven by your values is like making tea with such care that you add the tea leaves, sugar, and milk with your whole heart rather than just your hands. Habits become gentle affirmations that feed your spirit, speaking in the language of your ideals.

CHAPTER 1:
UNVEILING YOUR VALUES

The Essence and Impact of Values

Value is fundamentally like a jewel with several faces, each reflecting a particular hue, a different meaning, and a special significance to the viewer. Let's delicately dance through the numerous approaches and definitions illuminating its complex tapestry.

- **Economic Value:** A measure of how much a good or service is worth for other goods or services; economic value is frequently examined through utility, demand, and scarcity. The practical, observable value we attribute to objects greatly influences our daily interactions and economic choices.

- **Personal Value:** Personal values are the core of who we are, drifting towards the private spheres of our being. They serve as mild cues from our spirit that direct our deeds, choices, and encounters. Personal values, such as kindness, bravery, or integrity, are the colors with which we paint the picture of our lives.

- **Cultural Value:** A community or society is bound by its common beliefs and norms, called cultural values. The common comprehension of what is valued, revered, and honored shapes social relationships, customs, and shared stories.

- **Ethical and Moral Value:** Delving into the depths of philosophy, we now examine the inherent value of deeds, people, and things. Moral principles construct a road towards morally upright choices and acts by navigating the worlds of right and wrong, good and bad.

- **Aesthetic Value:** Exploring beauty in all manifestations, aesthetic value examines the inherent value in experiences, art, and the natural world. The soft prod causes us to stop and take in a sunset or lose ourselves in a song, enjoying beauty and expressiveness in their most basic forms.

Each facet of worth is like a window through which we can observe and engage with the environment. It's like having a compass built right into our heads, pointing the way through all the twists and turns of life.

All the different threads of your life—financial, cultural, ethical, and aesthetic—come together to form a tapestry that is uniquely and brilliantly you.

Let's pause for a bit as we carefully investigate values to allow our hearts and thoughts to gradually dip into a deeper reflection: What is the essence of a value? It's more than just a word or a conviction, but what sparks its vivacious, pulsing life within us?

Imagine a calm, peaceful pond reflecting the trees and sky surrounding it in a soft embrace. Value is fundamentally comparable in that it is a subdued representation of your inner landscape, reflecting your ingrained ideas, feelings, and sense of value and significance.

A value's essence can be found in its capacity to:

- **Guide:** Amid all the different roads that make up life's journey, the guide will softly illuminate your way.

- **Connect:** Creating a coherent, harmonious dance between your thoughts, feelings, and behaviors so that they sing a true, consistent tone.

- **Inspire:** Encouragement whispered into your spirit that inspires you to move, act, and make decisions by your innermost self.

A value's core skillfully weaves the intrinsic and extrinsic together into a rich tapestry that shapes our interior emotions and outward behaviors.

- **Intrinsic Essence:** Our intrinsic essence, which taps into the depths of our souls and resonates with our internal moral compass and emotional landscapes, inspires us to look within for meaning, purpose, and sincere contentment.

- **Extrinsic Essence:** This delicately touches on how we interact with the outside world—the behaviors, choices, and directions we make that are directly palpably shaped by our internal principles and shape our interpersonal connections, professional pathways, and social contributions.

If you go a little deeper, you'll discover that values have an energetic resonance that resonates with our sense of self, morality, and comprehension of the universe.

It's that emotional connection, the way a value can make us feel something, causing happiness or tranquility, or possibly discomfort or annoyance when our values are questioned or not upheld.

Now, imagine dropping a pebble into a calm body of water and watching the ripples become larger and larger as they softly cascade outward. Values behave similarly. Their initial effect is quiet, understated, barely a whisper. But how they spread, sending shockwaves into the world that cradles us and into our very existence.

1. Making Your Authentic Self a Priority

- Your values serve as an inner compass, delicately directing your thoughts, deeds, and choices.
- Living by your principles sows a deep, resonant fulfillment that nourishes the roots of pleasure and contentment.

- Values are strong anchors that help you stay anchored during turbulent times of transition and hardship.

2. Relational Impact: Stitching Genuine Connections Together

- Recognizing and respecting others' values creates a fertile environment where empathy and understanding can flourish.

- Building healthy relationships on a solid foundation of trust requires acting consistently from a position of value.

- Shared values frequently turn into the threads that weave people into a harmonious, cohesive tapestry, fostering a sense of belonging and harmony.

3. Social Impact: Creating Communities and Cultures

Social cohesion: In a society, shared values unite, bringing disparate people together around a common identity and goal.

Moral Framework: Values frequently shape society's moral and ethical framework by influencing rules, customs, and expectations.

Cultural Development: A society's ideals pervade its traditions, rituals, and culture, shaping and reflecting the people's collective spirit and character.

- By creating a global ethic that respects our common humanity, values like respect, empathy, and cooperation may direct international relations.
- Practices and policies that respect and safeguard our priceless planet are shaped by values like stewardship and responsibility.
- Promoting peace, resolving conflicts, and building peaceful inter-national coexistence among nations depend on universal principles like compassion, tolerance, and understanding.

Discovering Your Personal Values

Personal values, those intangible gems, are woven into the fabric of who you are. They gently yet firmly direct your actions, choices, and interactions. They are those steadfast torchbearers who shine a light on your path that aligns with your values and inner truths. Personal values are the many shades with which you paint your life's canvas, creating a painting that is honestly uniquely you. These shades range from kindness and integrity to ambition and curiosity.

Personal values have a profound and subtle power that resonates through the echo chambers of our existence, softly influencing how we live. They are the unseen builders who shape our lives, connections, and global impacts while building a legacy firmly founded in our core values. They impact the decisions we make, the relationships we form, and the pathways we decide to take, ensuring that each step chimes in tune with our true selves. When life's seas are choppy, personal values serve as our refuge, providing a solid foundation and a point of reference we can always rely on. They support our development and help us grow into mature individuals who can dance with life and manage it, expressing who we truly are.

Our values become a silent language that expresses who we are and what we stand for in interactions and relationships by delicately weaving threads of understanding and connection. They enable us to build connections based on respect and understanding for one another while navigating the web of human connection with sincerity and honesty. Honoring our principles gives us the freedom to live our lives as the most authentic versions of ourselves, creating relationships that accurately mirror our inner landscape. Here, in this wonderfully balanced existence, our values serve as a set of principles and as the foundation of who we are, influencing, reshaping, and giving our surroundings hues that truly represent who we are on the inside.

Imagine starting your journey by gently stepping into your personal experiences, reflections, and introspections. Explore the memories that brought you happiness, sorrow, frustration, or fulfillment. Dive into your past. Your values are frequently hidden but softly glimmering in the embers of those feelings and experiences, just waiting to be found. What has made you incredibly happy? When have you experienced intense anger or hurt? The answers to these questions frequently reveal what you value and cherish.

Connecting with your emotions can help you continue your journey since they are subtle signposts that lead to your values. Accept a thoughtful examination of your emotional responses to many circumstances, both in the past and the present. Investigate the reasons for your feelings. Frequently, when a circumstance makes you feel strongly, your values quietly whisper in your ear, giving you indications and cues about your innate ideas and principles.

Watch yourself now in action! Your actions and choices, particularly those taken on the spur of the moment, frequently reflect your values. Think about the decisions you've taken, the directions you've traveled, and the connections you've fostered. Your values are dancing there, showing themselves in your choices, conversations, and behaviors. Discover the principles that silently lead you by examining how your behaviors and deeply held beliefs line up.

Talk to yourself in the future for a moment. Imagine having a future perspective on yourself. What do you want to watch? What would fill you with pride, happiness, and fulfillment? Imagining the legacy and life story you want to leave behind may bring your ideals to light and direct your journey toward a destiny that resonates with your true self.

We sometimes see hints of our own ideals in the actions of others. Who inspires you, and why? What traits in other people appeal to you? The traits and values you appreciate in others frequently mirror your values, providing a lens through which you can examine and comprehend your guiding ideals.

Once you have gathered these shining pearls of values, take care of them since they are the seeds from which your true self will emerge. They need water from reflection, light from aware living, and room to grow. When they do, they will bloom and illuminate the way for you with their calm but steadfast presence.

You carry a road map created through reflection and investigation that directs you toward your ideals and true self. A journey towards a life that quietly resonates with the melody of your true being; each step on this route is a dance with your true self.

Reflections: Stories of Value Discovery

A Blank Canvas

Elara, a painter, turned to vivid colors and strokes to better convey her feelings. On a bright afternoon, she quietly contemplated why some colors spoke to her more than others as she viewed a canvas covered with them. The pastels conveyed a sense of softness, compassion, and tranquility to her, while the more vibrant colors conveyed strength, enthusiasm, and resolve. Elara understood that her paintings expressed her core beliefs: a delicate balance between calm and confidence. Every brushstroke became a silent dedication to the principles that subtly created her world, and her canvas became a reflection of her work and herself.

The Kind Cook

Chef Mia found her personal beliefs amid the hectic kitchen of a quaint downtown restaurant. The elderly customer who appreciated a dish that brought back fond memories of her late husband's cooking was the catalyst for her voyage of value discovery. Mia had a sudden epiphany: her cooking wasn't just a job but a vehicle for sharing her warmth, care, and compassion with the world. Her cooking was inspired by a desire to connect with others and share good food with those she cared about. Mia's profound culinary love was on full display as she converted the kitchen into a place where values of love, connection, and empathy simmered in every pot and pan.

The Conscious Gardener

Elias, a seasoned gardener, discovered that he could grow as a person amid flowers, trees, and soil. His garden was his sanctuary, where he could find solace and meaning amid nature. While tending to his plants one mild spring day, he saw a sapling struggling, its little leaves wilting in the hot heat. He carried it to a shady location and whispered words of comfort, assurance, and care. Elias realized that his gardening reflected his lifelong commitment to nurturing, safeguarding, and fostering development. He understood that he was a protector not just of plants but of all living things, providing them with loving attention and encouraging their development.

Each story's protagonist understood what was truly important to them through introspection, interpersonal experience, and habitual behavior. Mia discovered them in her culinary masterpieces and Elias in his loving care for all creatures, great and little. Each person came to their core beliefs through unique experiences and life journeys.

CHAPTER 2:
ANATOMY OF HABITS

How Habits are Formed: The Habit Loop

Habits are just routines we do repeatedly without even thinking about it. Think of them as well-traveled trails through the enchanted forest that is our life; the more we follow one, the clearer it becomes, and the easier it is to follow on subsequent visits. A habit develops from a single incident or "seed," firmly established in our routines and routine behaviors over time. The processes that drive our interpersonal relationships are just as much a habit as brushing our teeth every morning.

Look further into the craft of habits, and you'll see the extraordinary skill with which they shape our lives, carving out patterns and rhythms that echo through our being day in and day out. These unsaid, unseen patterns permeate every aspect of our lives, subtly but significantly reshaping our reality into the comfy shapes and rituals we rely on. The idea that our habits serve as unseen hands that shape and direct our lives is a beautiful metaphor that captures the delicate dance between our thoughts and deeds that is the fabric of our lives.

As you delve further, you'll see that our habits, in their quiet tenacity, become the artists of our character, revealing our core values and beliefs through our actions and decisions over time. We reveal our deepest, most personal ideals and the guiding principles by which we navigate life through our consistent, often unnoticed acts and decisions. We expose our true selves through the wordless language of routine action and behavior, which mirrors our inner reality as we nurture and cultivate habits.

However, the effects of habits are far-reaching, spreading like tendrils into our health and happiness, with the physical, emotional, and social dimensions all intertwined like tiles in a mosaic. The habits we develop, from caring for our bodies via mindful nutrition to caring for our souls through compassionate, sympathetic conversation, form a complex tapestry that subtly affects our health and happiness. Our actions, whether caring or neglectful, plant the seeds that will someday bear fruit in the form of our physical, mental, and social health, subtly steering our path toward harmony or discord.

Our habits appear as nebulous navigators in the whirlpool of decision-making, steering us with a light but steady hand. These unseen influences impact our daily journeys in both the literal and figurative senses, influencing our decisions and ensuring they are consistent with our habits and routines. Despite the frequently turbulent seas of life's decisions, our habits serve as steady, reliable guidance, acting as a compass that silently directs our course.

When developing expertise in a given field, our habits serve as unseen guides who help us persevere through the ups and downs of the arduous path to mastery. Consistent practice and committed improvement become the soil from which talents and competence emerge, whether through the melodic strings of an instrument or the savory excursions of culinary creations. Skills are sown in the soil of regular practice, where they flourish into the aromatic and musical threads of our lives that testify to our perseverance.

As we wind our way through the personal landscapes of our relationships, our habits entwine, becoming unseen but significant factors in how we relate to one another, express ourselves, and show affection. For our relationships to grow, flourish, and thrive in the rich, nurturing soil of true connection and care, the habits we cultivate—from sympathetic listening to sincere, passionate communication—are crucial. Our relationships flourish into dynamic manifestations of mutual respect, understanding, and love when we cultivate them via habits of the heart and soul.

An intriguing aspect is that habits can serve as both builders and confinement. They can help us build a life full of health, happiness, and harmony, or they can stifle us if we let them take the form of harmful or unhealthy routines. To reap the benefits and minimize the drawbacks of our habits, we must first become aware of them, analyze them, and then consciously shape them.

Influences and Impact of Habits

Our habits, the little things we do repeatedly without giving them much thought, have a surprisingly large influence on who we are and how we live. Let's look into the power of habit formation and its far-reaching consequences.

Habit-Forming Factors

Our environment is a major factor in determining our behaviors. Our environments, including our homes, workplaces, and recreational haunts, can facilitate or sabotage our efforts to form positive routines. A messy desk might be distracting, whereas access to a gym can motivate you to exercise regularly.

People we associate with have a substantial effect on our behavior. The people in our lives can encourage us to stick to healthy routines or discourage us from doing so. Our social groups can either support us or test our beliefs and habits.

Habits can be greatly influenced by the structure and regularity of our daily routines. Creating a routine in our daily lives can help us more easily adopt new, positive behaviors. Conversely, it can be not easy to maintain new behaviors if they aren't established regularly.

Our emotional state can influence our behavior. Overeating and smoking are two bad coping mechanisms that may result from stress, while engaging in physical activity and mindfulness meditation may be beneficial.

Effects of Regular Behavior

Our habits can majorly affect both of these factors. Productivity can be increased by adopting constructive routines, such as goal-setting and time management, while stagnation can be caused by procrastination.

One of the most obvious ways in which our habits affect our lives is through the state of our health and wellness. Our physical and mental health is directly impacted by our dietary and lifestyle choices and our ability to deal with stress. On the contrary, engaging in harmful behaviors might shorten one's life expectancy and diminish one's energy.

Personal Development and Growth. Habits play a significant role in both. For example, making it a practice to always be learning new things can help you develop personally and professionally. Creating routines of introspection and objective setting can also be beneficial to development.

The quality of our interpersonal connections is impacted by our routines. Relationships thrive when people make it a habit to listen attentively, show compassion, and talk to one another. Conversely, bad habits like lying or being passive-aggressive can cause friction and damage trust in interpersonal connections.

Prosperity monetarily. Our financial security is directly tied to our spending patterns. Positive financial habits that can lead to financial stability include sticking to a budget, saving money, and investing, whereas negative habits that can lead to financial stress include spending more than you earn and accruing debt.

Habits are the link between goal-setting and actual success. Consistent and goal-oriented habits help us move closer to our dreams and bring us closer to realizing our ambitions.

Mindfulness, gratitude, and stress reduction are all practices that can positively affect our mental health. With these practices, we may face and overcome obstacles confidently and optimistically.

The Power and Pitfalls of Habituation

The process through which a person's brain becomes accustomed to a stimulus through repeated exposure is called habituation. It's neat at first because it lets you zero down on fresh and interesting things. Let's say you have to live next to a really noisy street. After a while, your brain will be like, "Meh, heard it all before," and you won't notice the traffic noise anymore.

The drawback is that routine can cause you to overlook critical details. When you're used to something, it's easy to miss changes or threats. It's like having a noisy clock in your room; after a while, you don't even notice when the time starts to move erratically.

And it's not all about the goods you own. Even with feelings, this can occur. Your upbeat disposition could become the new standard for you. When something truly remarkable occurs, though, you may not react with the enthusiasm it merits since your mind tells you, "Eh, it's just another day."

While habituation might help you enjoy the novel and be exciting, it can also dull your senses to the important and make you take the wonderful things in life for granted. Friend, it cuts both ways.

Let's explore the dangers of habituation together, buddy. It's like a stealthy ninja that can catch you off guard.

Missed Details

Consider that the painting you hold in the highest esteem is on your wall. You see it every day, and it makes you happy, makes you feel secure, and gives you motivation. A small, barely noticeable tear has appeared in the corner of the canvas.

After a while, you stop seeing this picture because "Oh, it's just part of the scenery," which means that you see it so regularly that it has become second nature. Day after day, the rip worsens as you go about your daily routine. As dust accumulates, it becomes more difficult to fix.

The harmful effects of habituation become apparent now. It would help if you had repaired that tear when it was only a minor annoyance. That minor rip has grown into a huge tear because you either didn't notice it or didn't believe it was a big concern. It's no longer a minor problem but rather a serious one that will necessitate more time, energy, and resources to fix.

More than only paintings are involved. It's about how you can become so used to something that you fail to see any changes or problems with it. It might be an odd noise from your car, a gradual decline in your health, or strained relationships. Getting used to these shifts or difficulties increases the likelihood that you won't handle them when they're still manageable, escalating a much larger, messier issue.

Emotional Flatline

Imagine you're in a relationship that initially filled you with unimaginable happiness. You grin when you open your eyes next to your loved one every morning, and the world around you is like a soft, comforting blanket. You find it incredibly reassuring and wonderful.

However, this is where familiarity sets in. The initial zeal and enthusiasm gradually wane with time. Things that used to make you feel warm and fuzzy inside have become boring or even expected. You have been accustomed to being happy, and thus, the gradual shift toward discontent may pass you by at first.

You and your partner may become emotionally distant or argue more frequently. There's a slight change in the atmosphere, as when a storm is just beginning to gather on the horizon, but you don't notice it. You've grown accustomed to being happy in this partnership and don't want to risk spoiling things by making a major change.

The catch is there. You've become accustomed to this "meh" condition and are coasting along happily, oblivious to the fact that things are actually getting worse behind the scenes. What previously made you feel complete is slowly fading away. When you could be working to nourish and rejuvenate your relationship, you're instead locked in a comfortable but stagnant routine.

Relationships aren't the only place where people experience emotional flatlining. Perhaps you've gotten so used to the security of your employment that you're oblivious that it's losing its luster. You may be too comfortable in a routine that no longer provides a worthwhile challenge or sense of adventure.

Boredom

Consider the music that has meant the most to you. The song that causes you to instantly start dancing whenever you hear it. It's so good that you keep listening to it repeatedly. An initial surge of vitality, a musical equivalent of a shot of adrenaline. However, an intriguing phenomenon occurs as the weeks progress into the months.

The power of that song, which used to make you feel better instantly, gradually faded away. It's not that the tune has suddenly changed; it's still the same stunning tune that won your heart. It's on the inside where the shift occurs. Your ingenious brain has already begun to tune out the music. They're thinking, "Oh, this again?" Yawn."

You suddenly realize that the song you used to blast has faded into the background. The feelings and enthusiasm it once inspired are no longer present. It's become ordinary; there's nothing remarkable about it.

Now, this has nothing to do with music alone. It applies to any situation in which you go overboard. Excessive repetition can make even the most exciting experiences boring. The thrill of your go-to pastime, the allure of your favorite TV show, or the allure of your ideal holiday site can fade if you spend too much time there.

The lesson here is that having options is important. Even the most thrilling adventures can become mundane after enough repetition. Trying new things, taking up new hobbies, and occasionally stretching one's comfort zone are all great ways to keep life interesting and exciting.

Stuck in a Rut

Habits are like the cozy slippers you want to wear after a long day. They're simple, reassuring, and comfortable to fall back on. After all, who doesn't enjoy a cuddly sensation of contentment now and then?

Those cozy slippers are great, but here's the deal: they may also serve as a metaphor for how habits operate in our lives. It's as comfortable as wearing those slippers all the time when you keep doing the same things over and over again. It's wonderful and relaxing, but you can lose out on life outside your comfort zone.

Let's use the example of having the same bowl of cereal every morning. It's comforting to the palate and requires little effort on your part. What, though? A wide variety of breakfast foods is available for your perusal, from light pancakes to hearty omelets.

Habitually repeating the same boring activities might be as unsatisfying as eating the same breakfast cereal every day. Suppose you stick to the same pattern daily. In that case, you risk becoming bored and missing out on life's varied and interesting experiences. Imagine having a treasure box full of exciting events, possibilities, and adventures but sticking with the same old key.

Please don't misunderstand me; routines really are that important. They provide us a sense of stability, predictability, and security. But when they become too set in stone and unyielding, they can prohibit you from exploring the entire breadth of what life has to offer.

Missing Out on Growth

Think about it: there's a restaurant that offers your favorite meal of all time. You know that dish will be wonderful, so order it whenever you go there. It's safe, it's known, and it never fails to satisfy.

There's certainly nothing wrong with having a go-to food; the comfort of eating something you know and love never fails to satisfy. But now we come to the crux of the matter. You always stick to the same food since you've grown accustomed to it. You don't give the remainder of the menu, which is filled with interesting and unusual dishes, a second thought.

Food symbolizes life, not just a means to an end. It's easy to avoid trying new things when stuck in a rut of old routines and habits. Like returning to a tried-and-true favorite cuisine, doing so provides a sense of security and familiarity. But that would mean missing out on life's rich, varied, and often spicy flavors.

Whether it's sampling a new dish, picking up a new talent, or visiting a new location, every new experience enriches the rich fabric of your life. It's like spicing up your meal with a pinch of something new and interesting; it stimulates your senses, makes you think critically, and broadens your horizons.

Consider this. You must venture outside your comfort zone to feel the thrill of discovery. You won't be able to develop personally or intellectually. Instead of a symphony of lovely and varied music, life might start to sound like a monotone anthem.

CHAPTER 3: DESIGNING YOUR VALUE-INFUSED HABITS

Strategies to Formulate Habits Aligned with Values

Prioritize Your Values

Think of your values as a collection of rare diamonds, each one special and priceless in its own right. Your decisions are influenced by these values, which also help to characterize you and determine how your life will pan out. However, the relevance of your values might vary, just as not all stones are the same rarity or value.

Organizing your values according to importance is similar to sorting these diamonds to determine which ones in your life's mosaic shine the brightest. Here's why it's so important:

1. Clarity in Decision-Making: When faced with options or conundrums, prioritizing your values gives you clarity. You may make choices supporting your top priorities when you know which values are most important. It's similar to having a compass that consistently directs you in the proper path.
2. Resource Allocation: You have limited time, energy, and resources. You can distribute these limited resources more wisely

by determining and prioritizing your values. You'll put more money into the principles that are important to you and are most likely to improve your life.

3. Put Your Attention on What Really Matters: Not all values are created equal, and some may have more personal significance for you than others. Setting your values in order will help you concentrate on what is most important to you. Making a deliberate decision to focus your efforts where they will have the biggest impact.

4. Overcoming Value Conflicts: Values occasionally clash with one another. For instance, your value of work-life balance can be at odds with your value of job success. You can resolve these conflicts through prioritization by determining which value should take precedence in a certain circumstance.

5. Achieving Greater Fulfillment: You have a stronger feeling of fulfillment and purpose when your behaviors align with your highest priority values. Living following what most closely aligns with who you truly are might increase overall contentment.

Here is a useful method to order your values:

1. Identify Your Values: List all the values that matter to you. Honesty, compassion, family, professional achievement, personal development, adventure, and many more are examples.

2. examine Significance: Give each value some thought and examine its importance in your life. You should ask yourself such things as "How much does this value matter to me?" and "How does this value influence my choices and actions?"

3. Group and Rank: Compile related values into a single group before ranking them according to importance. Some values may naturally cluster, which can make it easier for you to spot overarching trends.

4. Think About Personal Goals: Consider your immediate and long-term objectives. Which principles best support these objectives? Setting values that support your objectives as priorities might show you the way forward.

5. Conduct Regular Reviews: Values may change over time. Review your values periodically to make sure they still reflect your ideas and objectives. Set new priorities as necessary.

You might think of prioritizing your values as building a hierarchy that directs your daily decisions and habit formation. The habits you develop will clearly represent your values thanks to this hierarchy, which will ultimately result in a more meaningful and genuine life journey.

Create a Habit Loop

Think of your values as a collection of rare diamonds, each one special and priceless in its own right. Your decisions are influenced by these values, which also help to characterize you and determine how your life will pan out. However, the relevance of your values might vary, just as not all stones are the same rarity or value.

Organizing your values according to importance is similar to sorting these diamonds to determine which ones in your life's mosaic shine the brightest. Here's why it's so important:

1. Clarity in Decision-Making: When faced with options or conundrums, prioritizing your values gives you clarity. You may make choices supporting your top priorities when you know which values are most important. It's similar to having a compass that consistently directs you in the proper path.

2. Resource Allocation: You have limited time, energy, and resources. You can distribute these limited resources more wisely by determining and prioritizing your values. You'll put more money into the principles that are important to you and are most likely to improve your life.

3. Put Your Attention on What Really Matters: Not all values are created equal, and some may have more personal significance for you than others. Setting your values in order will help you concentrate on what is most important to you. Making a deliberate decision to focus your efforts where they will have the biggest impact.

4. Overcoming Value Conflicts: Values might occasionally clash with one another. For instance, your value of work-life balance can be at odds with your value of job success. You can resolve these conflicts through prioritization by determining which value should take precedence in a certain circumstance.

5. Achieving Greater Fulfillment: You have a stronger feeling of fulfillment and purpose when your behaviors align with your highest priority values. Living by what most closely aligns with who you truly are might increase overall contentment.

Here is a useful method to order your values:

1. Identify Your Values: List all the values that matter to you. Honesty, compassion, family, professional achievement, personal development, adventure, and many more are examples.

2. Examine the Significance: Give each value some thought and examine its importance in your life. You should ask yourself such things as "How much does this value matter to me?" and "How does this value influence my choices and actions?"

3. Group and Rank: Compile related values into a single group before ranking them according to importance. Some values may naturally cluster, which can make it easier for you to spot overarching trends.

4. Think About Personal Goals: Consider your immediate and long-term objectives. Which principles best support these objectives? Setting values that support your objectives as priorities might show you the way forward.

5. Conduct Regular Reviews: Values may change over time. Review your values periodically to make sure they still reflect your ideas and objectives. Set new priorities as necessary.

You might think of prioritizing your values as building a hierarchy that directs your daily decisions and habit formation. The habits you develop will clearly represent your values thanks to this hierarchy, which will ultimately result in a more meaningful and genuine life journey.

Track your Progress

Keeping a record of your progress keeps you on the correct track and gives you a concrete record of your accomplishments, much like having a map on your road to habit development. Let's look at why tracking is important and how it can have a big impact on your habit-building process:

1. Responsibility:

Imagine yourself traveling across the country by car. Despite having a certain destination, you risk getting lost or taking unneeded diversions if you need a map or GPS. Comparably, tracking your progress when forming a new habit is your GPS, holding you responsible and ensuring you stay on target.

You develop a sense of accountability for yourself by recording your daily or weekly efforts in a journal or utilizing a habit-tracking app. You can observe if you're steadily progressing toward your objective or getting off course. You are encouraged to keep going and make modifications as needed by being conscious of your progress.

2. Imagination:

It's like watching a movie about your development as your habit-building adventure plays out. It gives you a visual depiction of your advancement, which may be inspiring. It is comparable to glancing at the mileage on your trip's route map.

Track your behaviors as a visual chronology of your efforts. When you reflect on your past, you can see patterns of stability, successful streaks, and potential places for growth. You can see the results of your actions and the steady transformation that is occurring with the aid of this visualization.

3. Motivation & Encouragement:

Take a hike up a challenging mountain. It's difficult, and occasionally you feel worn out and ready to give up. But when you regularly pause and consider how far you've come, it serves as a reminder of your accomplishments and a motivation to keep moving forward.

Keeping track of your habit-forming progress has a comparable benefit. When you can see that your efforts are impacting, it provides moments of inspiration and motivation. Even minor successes or the straightforward act of keeping a streak going might give you more self-assurance and motivation.

4. Modifications and Learning:

Tracking involves not only recognizing accomplishments but also taking lessons from failures. Your tracking record might be a great resource should you run into problems or need to remember a day when forming a habit.

You can assess the circumstances that contributed to your error, including any mental or behavioral issues or a lack of preparation. You may make the required adjustments and create strategies to deal with problems in the future with the aid of this reflective process. It's similar to looking for alternate routes on your road trip map when the main road is blocked.

5. Long-Term Outlook:

A marathon, not a sprint, is required to create new habits. In the thick of the daily grind, losing sight of your long-term objectives can take time and effort. Monitoring your development is a compass to keep you pointed toward the greater vision.

The cumulative effect of your efforts can be shown by keeping a record over time. It serves as a reminder that every day and every action advances the main objective. It's similar to placing waypoints on your road trip map to indicate the paths you've already traveled and those still in front of you.

Learn from Setbacks

A vital component of habit-building and personal development is learning from failures. It's similar to running into barriers and detours while traveling; rather than giving up, you take advantage of these obstacles as chances to improve as a traveler on the path to success. Here's why it's so important to view failures as teaching opportunities:

1. Accepting Setbacks:

The first and most important thing to understand is that setbacks are a necessary component of the habit-building process. Very few people start a new habit journey without running into challenges. You're less likely to get discouraged when failures arise if you anticipate them.

2. Adaptation and Resilience:

The opportunity to develop resilience and adaptation is presented by setbacks. Imagine them like the weather you experience when traveling. It might sometimes be bright and easygoing, or it can be tough and stormy. When you overcome obstacles, you get the fortitude to face challenges and the versatility to change your tactics.

3. Examining the Causes:

Setbacks allow you to explore the "why" behind your difficulties. Was your routine disrupted by outside events or internal struggles like a lack of drive or self-control? You can proactively deal with difficulties by understanding what might cause them in the future by evaluating the underlying causes of setbacks.

4. Refining Techniques:

Setbacks warn that your present strategy may need to be modified. They encourage you to contemplate "What can I do differently?" and "How can I overcome this challenge?" This process of reflection might help you develop better tactics and have a deeper understanding of what works for you.

5. Strengthening Persistence:

Overcoming obstacles strengthens one's capacity for perseverance. You strengthen your resolve and devotion each time you overcome a setback and keep working toward your habit. This tenacity is an important quality you may use in various aspects of your life besides habit-building.

6. Honoring Minor Victories:

Celebrating the large and minor wins along the way to breaking bad habits is important. No matter how modest, overcoming a setback is cause for celebration. It confirms your development and reminds you that you may overcome obstacles.

7. Change in Attitude:

Consider setbacks as stepping stones on your journey to success rather than failures. Thanks to this mentality shift, you can embrace setbacks with curiosity and a growth-oriented viewpoint. Setbacks lose their ability to demotivate you when you change your attention from failing to learning.

8. Personal Development:

In the end, failures help you develop personally. They push you to change, adapt, and learn new things. You develop resiliency, creativity, and knowledge whenever you encounter and overcome a setback.

9. Sustainability through time:

Building habits involves making long-lasting changes, not merely accomplishing a short-term objective. The ability to continuously improve and modify your habits to meet your changing circumstances and values ensures that your habits are sustainable.

In conclusion, setbacks are not obstacles but rather stepping stones on your path to developing values-aligned behaviors. Accept them as chances for development, education, and advancement. You may turn losses into important lessons that advance you toward your goals and ideals by assessing setbacks, improving your tactics, and keeping a growth-oriented mindset.

Flexibility and Adaptation

You may fly through life's dynamic and constantly changing terrain with the help of flexibility and adaptation, which are like your wings. You can use flexibility to ensure your routines align with your changing values and circumstances, much as a bird modifies its flight path to navigate shifting winds and weather conditions. Here are some reasons why adaptability is a key component in the art of habit formation:

1. Recognizing the dynamic nature of life:

Life is a dynamic, always-changing experience rather than a still, unchanging journey. Opportunities, difficulties, and experiences keep coming up. Recognizing this dynamic nature helps you realize how important it is for your habits to be flexible to account for these changes.

2. Adhering to Changing Values:

Your values can grow and develop through time; they are not fixed in stone. Your values may change as you mature and gain new understanding, causing you to give certain parts of your life more weight. You can modify your habits to reflect these changing values if you are flexible.

3. Adjusting to Changing Conditions:

Unexpected setbacks are a common part of life. Your circumstances can drastically change due to a job change, the addition of a new family member, or a move. Flexible habits can be altered to fit your new reality, like a well-tailored suit, ensuring they continue to be applicable and realistic.

4. Avoiding Stability:

Rigid routines might keep you stuck in a rut and give you the impression that you are being held captive. Your routines are given new life through flexibility, which keeps them from getting boring or heavy.

5. Positivity in the Face of Difficulties:

There will always be obstacles and failures. Flexible habits can adjust to accommodate challenges, making them resilient. Setbacks don't stop you from moving forward; they provide growth and course adjustment opportunities.

6. Development of Sustainable Habits:

Flexible habits are more likely to last over time. Because they are flexible, they are less prone to generate fatigue or frustration. For you to continue progressing and accomplishing your objectives, sustainability is essential.

7. Supporting Diversification and Exploration

The path to variety and discovery is opened by flexibility. It enables you to experiment with new methods, test various tactics, and bring creativity into daily routines. This makes your journey interesting and encourages curiosity.

8. Promoting Learning and Growth:

A type of growth in itself is altering your routines to reflect shifting circumstances and ideals. It supports lifelong learning and personal growth. You develop greater flexibility and resourcefulness, enabling you to handle life's challenges with grace and resiliency.

9. Creating an Individualized Lifestyle:

In the end, flexibility enables you to design a lifestyle that is specifically catered to you. Curating habits that reflect your values is a conscious decision, but it also acknowledges that these habits will need to change and adapt as your life story develops.

Flexibility can be included in habit formation without sacrificing commitment or consistency. Instead, it entails accepting change as a necessary component of your path and changing your routines accordingly. It's about keeping your mind open to new ideas, following your inner compass, and ensuring your habits still support your quest for a life rooted in your highest ideals. You may successfully manage the ever-changing life currents while adhering to your basic values and objectives when flexible.

Common Challenges and Solutions in Habit Design

Creating and establishing new routines may be an interesting and challenging adventure. To assist you in overcoming these obstacles, let's look at some typical difficulties encountered when designing habits and some efficient approaches to overcoming them.

Lack of Motivation

A lack of motivation is one of the most frequent obstacles to the need for more new habits. It's similar to the initial rush of excitement at the starting line of a race, only to struggle to hold onto that zeal as you move forward. Here is a more thorough investigation of this issue and practical strategies to keep your motivation strong:

Challenge: The Motivational Flame Is Waning

You frequently feel a motivational high at the start of your habit-forming journey. You're enthusiastic, motivated by the possibility of making a difference, and eager to start your new habit. However, as time goes on, that initial spark may fade, resulting in a lack of momentum and making it challenging to continue your practices consistently.

Option 1: Establish definite objectives

Think of your drive like a ship sailing a big ocean. The North Star of clear objectives will point your ship on the right path even in rough seas. Setting specific goals will help you regain your motivation in the following ways:

Specificity: Clearly state the goals you have for your habit. Ensure your objectives are SMART—specific, measurable, achievable, relevant, and time-bound. For instance, if you routinely work out, a SMART goal may be, "I will go for a 30-minute jog every morning at 6 AM."

Tracking Progress: Goals give you a way to gauge your development. Measurable advancements strengthen your sense of accomplishment and keep you engaged. It's similar to placing waypoints on a map as you go toward your destination.

Sense of Purpose: Clear objectives link your habit to a bigger cause, giving it a sense of purpose. They serve as a reminder of your original motivation for starting this adventure. Your behaviors will become more intrinsic and persistent when rooted in purpose.

Option 2: Look for Internal Motivation

The fuel that stokes the fire within is intrinsic motivation. It acts as your internal engine to carry you on when the influence of outside forces wanes. How to use intrinsic motivation is as follows:

Align with Values: Establish a link between your behavior and fundamental principles. For instance, if you believe in the importance of health and well-being, remind yourself how your workout routine supports these beliefs. Your activities have more meaning when they are consistent with your values.

Intrinsic Reward: Look for rewards that are unique to the habit. Engage in your habit with joy, contentment, or a sense of success.

It's similar to enjoying the journey rather than only focusing on the end goal.

Mindful Presence: Being mindfully present is being fully involved with your habit. You can access the inherent happiness of the present when you fully engage in the experience. It's similar to enjoying every mouthful of a wonderful meal and taking pleasure in the journey rather than simply the destination.

Option 3: Envision Success

Think of motivation as a fire that occasionally has to be stoked to remain bright. Adding logs to a fire is analogous to visualization. Here's how it might spark your excitement once more:

Create a Mental Blueprint: Create a mental blueprint by regularly visualizing yourself carrying out your habit successfully. Think about the satisfying results and your own sense of achievement. This mental map can serve as a strong motivator.

Good associations: Connect your habit with good feelings and associations through imagination. You're more likely to approach your habit enthusiastically if you associate it with feelings of joy, pride, or contentment.

Future Reward: Consider the advantages and rewards your habit will provide in the long run. It can be quite motivating to picture yourself as healthier, happier, and more content.

To effectively combat the problem of dwindling motivation, it is important to understand the deeper significance of your habits, set specific goals to give you direction, and use visualization to stoke your passion. You can maintain the flame of inspiration throughout your quest for significant change by including these solutions in your habit-forming journey.

Overwhelm

On your path to habit building, overwhelm can be a terrible foe. It's comparable to juggling twelve balls at once after only learning to juggle three. This problem sometimes appears when you try to build too many new behaviors at once and bite off more than you can chew. Take into account the following ways to overcome this difficulty and guarantee that your habit-forming efforts are moderate and long-lasting:

Overwhelm—Floundering in a Sea of Ambitions

Adopting many new habits at once is tempting when you're motivated to make great improvements in several areas of your life. However, this energy can easily become exhaustion, drowning you in a sea of commitments and desires.

Option 1: Begin Minimally

Think about forming habits as foundational elements. Laying a strong foundation for your habit structure by starting small is similar. Here's why this strategy works so well:

Manageable Steps: Include one or two realistically achievable behaviors into your daily or weekly schedule. These routines should not be difficult to maintain. For instance, starting with a daily 10-minute walk rather than committing to a daily one-hour workout is a more realistic first step if your goal is to increase your fitness.

Gain Confidence: Succeeding in modest habits increases your self-assurance and faith in your ability to adopt new habits. Every accomplishment acts as a springboard for bigger transformations. It's comparable to gradually increasing the weight of a barbell as your strength increases.

Focus and Consistency: You can better focus your energy and attention by focusing on several habits. This sharpened focus enables you to build a solid foundation of consistency, which is essential for creating long-lasting habits.

Option 2: Create a habit hierarchy

Imagine a forest of trees representing your behaviors. Making a habit hierarchy is similar to picking out and focusing on the biggest, tallest trees first. Prioritization can help with the following:

Clarifying Importance: Consider each habit's importance in light of your overall life objectives. Which behaviors most significantly affect your well-being or are most consistent with your values? Put these habits first since they will pay the biggest dividends on your investment.

Spreading Your Efforts Too Thin: By creating a habit hierarchy, you can avoid spreading your efforts too widely across various behaviors. By concentrating on them first, you should allocate enough time and effort to build the most crucial ones.

Progressive Expansion: Once your top priorities are well-defined, you may add new behaviors gradually while building on the foundation you've already constructed. This systematic approach reduces the possibility of feeling overburdened and makes it easier to adjust to new routines.

In conclusion, overcoming the overload difficulty requires understanding the limitations of handling too much at once. You may overcome the difficulties of habit formation by beginning small and developing a habit hierarchy. This will also ensure that each habit you develop has a chance to take hold and flourish. This strategy prepares the road for a successful habit-formation journey consistent with your beliefs and goals.

Lack of Accountability

Being unreliable might be likened to navigating a ship without a compass or a navigator. When no one keeps track of your progress, going off course is simple, and keeping your routines consistent becomes difficult. Consider the following strategies to overcome this difficulty and make sure you continue on your path to habit formation:

Problem: Navigating the Waters of Habit Formation Alone in The Lone Sailor's Dilemma

Without external checks and balances, it's simple to get lost or lose enthusiasm when starting a habit-forming journey alone.

Option 1: Accountability Partners

Think of your accountability partners as your fellow captains on the habit-forming ship. How they can help you succeed is as follows:

Shared Commitment: Tell a friend, family member, or coworker whom you can trust about your goals and desired behaviors. There is an inherent sense of accountability to someone when they are aware of your objectives.

Regular Check-Ins: Plan frequent check-in meetings with your accountability partner to go through your progress. You may be inspired to maintain consistency if you know someone is following your progress.

Mutual Support: A supportive and encouraging accountability partner is a valuable resource. You can mutually encourage one another's efforts to build habits by exchanging advice and rejoicing over victories.

Option 2: Use habit-tracking

Apps for habit tracking serve as your digital compass and diary. Your habit-forming path is given structure and accountability by them:

Record and Monitor: Real-time tracking of your daily or weekly progress is possible with these apps. Tracking helps you stay committed to your habits, and observing your streaks may be inspiring.

Visual Feedback: Numerous habit-tracking apps provide visual feedback through calendars or charts to show your development. It's simple to see how consistent you've been with these visualizations, which may motivate you to continue your streak.

Create Reminders: These apps frequently have reminder capabilities that remind you to practice your habit at predetermined periods or times. Even when life gets hectic, reminders can help you keep up with your routine.

Option 3: Public Commitment

Making a public pledge is similar to flying your ship's flag. It makes your intentions known to the public, which makes it harder to veer from your chosen path.

Share on Social Media: Consider posting about your habit development on social media sites. A strong sense of external accountability might be derived from knowing that people know your intentions.

Join a Group: You can interact with like-minded people by taking part in local or online habit development communities. These groups frequently provide assistance, inspiration, and a forum for discussing development.

Challenges for Accountability: Set up contests or challenges with friends or online communities. A strong motivator can be the desire to perform better than others or the fear of failing.

In conclusion, overcoming the lack of accountability entails utilizing other sources of assistance and supervision to assist you in maintaining your routines. These solutions provide the checks and balances necessary to successfully traverse the occasionally turbulent waters of habit development through accountability partners, habit-tracking applications, or public commitment. You can steer a steady course toward the habits and values you want to adopt if you have the correct support system.

Resistance Change

It can feel like you're trying to shift a huge boulder firmly planted in your way when you encounter resistance to change. Because we are creatures of habit, changing from our regular routines can be difficult and uncomfortable. Consider these strategies to handle this issue and successfully negotiate the challenging terrain of habit change:

Challenge: Pushing Your Inner Self to Embrace Change Despite the Comfort of Familiarity
Resistance is frequently sparked by the idea of change because it threatens the regularity and comfort of long-standing routines.

Option 1: Gradual Transition

Think of changing your habits as stepping stones across a river. The stepping stones that make the path easier and less intimidating are provided by gradual change. This is how it goes:

Progressive Steps: If your desired habit would require a big change to your daily routine, divide it into more doable, smaller steps. For instance, if you want to meditate every day, start with just a few minutes a day and build up to longer sessions.

Incremental Changes: You can lessen the impact of an abrupt shift by making minor, gradual changes to your daily routine. It's similar to gradually acclimating to a new environment so that your comfort zone can grow at a controllable rate.

Consolidate Gains: Gains should be built upon when you successfully implement one minor modification by adding the next one. This technique lets you gradually develop your desired habit by accumulating minor victories.

Option 2: Practice self-compassion

Offering oneself self-compassion is similar to giving yourself a soothing salve to lessen the pain of transformation. This is why it's essential:

Recognize Discomfort: Accept that discomfort is a normal component of change. Similar to how your muscles hurt after a new workout, this is a sign that you are evolving and expanding.

Develop Patience: Recognize that habit change is a process and that making mistakes along the way is acceptable. Be kind and patient with yourself as you make your way through the new region of change, just as you wouldn't chastise a toddler learning to walk for falling down.

Replace Self-Criticism: Use self-compassion instead of punishing oneself for mistakes or failures. Give yourself the same consideration and support you would extend to a friend in a similar situation.

Positive Self-Talk: Use positive affirmations and self-talk to strengthen your will to change. Remember why you want to develop the habit and the advantages it will have for you.

In conclusion, overcoming reluctance to change requires realizing that your comfort zone is like a cocoon—a secure and comfortable environment. Your skills for gently encouraging your inner self to accept change are gradual transition and self-compassion. You may overcome the discomfort and reluctance that frequently come with changing your habits by breaking the change down into manageable steps and treating yourself with kindness and patience. Doing this will open the door for long-lasting change that reflects your beliefs and goals.

Inconsistency

Consistency is comparable to constructing a sandcastle while the tide keeps flowing in and destroying your efforts. It's a typical obstacle in habit building because life's unpredictability may easily derail even the best-laid plans. Consider these strategies to overcome this difficulty and keep up the continuous momentum required for habit formation:

Challenge: Consistency's Ebb and Flow

The foundation for creating new habits is consistency. Habits are formed by daily or frequent repetition, yet even the most diligent routines can be disturbed by the unpredictable nature of life.

Option 1: Create a setback plan

Consider the journey of your habits as a strenuous walk. Planning for setbacks is similar to bringing the necessary equipment to tackle unforeseen roadblocks. Here's why this strategy is essential:

Identify Potential barriers: Be aware of any barriers or problems preventing you from maintaining your habit. These could consist of unforeseen circumstances, family obligations, or work deadlines.

Create backup plans: Have a backup plan for each potential hiccup. This strategy can entail altering your habit's practice schedule, developing alternate methods, or admitting that some days require flexibility.

Keep Your Adaptability: Habit formation requires changing with the environment. You are less likely to become frustrated when life throws you curveballs if you prepare for setbacks and are adaptable.

Option 2: Forgive yourself

Consider consistency to be a marathon. It's common to stumble or briefly lag behind in this race. Self-forgiveness practice is similar to getting back up and finishing the marathon with renewed vigor. Why this strategy is crucial is as follows:

Recognize Imperfection: Recognize that mistakes and missed days are a normal part of the habit-forming process and that no one is perfect. They don't determine your growth; how you handle them counts.

Focus on the Present: Refocus on the present moment rather than lingering on past mistakes or feeling guilty. Every day presents a chance to reconfirm your dedication to your habit.

Learn from Setbacks: Consider setbacks as chances for development. Examine what went wrong and think of ways to prevent it from happening again. Setbacks are turned into worthwhile lessons through this reflecting process.

Keep a Growth attitude: Adopt a growth attitude that recognizes that setbacks are transient and that progress is a journey containing both highs and lows. Your persistence and adaptability are evidence of your development.

In conclusion, dealing with the problem of consistency requires accepting that life is unpredictable and that failures are a typical part of the habit-forming process. You can overcome these difficulties with resilience and grace by planning for setbacks and engaging in self-forgiveness exercises. Doing this ensures that little slip-ups uphold your overall development and maintain your long-term commitment to your routines and ideals.

Activities: Crafting Your Initial Habit Designs

Making your early habit designs can be a creative and reflective process that prepares you for the habit-forming process. Here is a simple exercise to get you started:

Supplies required:

- A diary or notepad
- pens, pencils, markers, or any other preferred writing or drawing instruments

Step 1: Reflect on Your Values and Objectives (15 minutes)

To write in your journal, find a quiet and welcoming place. Consider your principles and overarching life goals for a moment. What is most important to you? Do you picture the kind of life you want for yourself?

Step 2: Determine Your Priorities (15 minutes)

Using your beliefs and goals as a guide, list your top priorities. These could fall under headings like "health," "relationships," "personal development," "career," or "leisure." Be clear and sincere with yourself about what is genuinely important to you at this time.

Step 3: Spend 15 minutes coming up with habit ideas (15 minutes)

Create a list of habit ideas consistent with your values and objectives for each priority. At this point, don't worry about viability or practicality; concentrate on coming up with as many ideas as possible. If "health" is a priority, habit suggestions can include daily exercise, drinking more water, or consuming more veggies.

Step 4: Limit Your Options (10 minutes)

Review your list of potential habits and mark the ones that most speak to you. You are most eager and motivated to pursue these habits. Especially if you're new to habit building, try to pick one or two habits.

Step 5: Define Your Habits (15 minutes)

Define each habit you choose in detail and detail. Create a brief habit statement using the SMART criteria: Specific, Measurable, Achievable, Relevant, and Time-bound. If you exercise regularly, you may define your habit as "I will go for a 30-minute walk every morning at 7 AM."

Step 6: Create a Habit Plan (10 minutes)

Create a plan now for each habit. Determine the times and locations where you will practice the habit, any required tools or resources, and how you will get through any challenges. Your road map for creating new habits is this one.

Step 7: Envision Success (10 minutes)

Put your eyes closed and inhale deeply a few times. Imaginc yourself successfully implementing the habits you've chosen. Consider the advantages these behaviors will bring to your life. You can increase your motivation and dedication by visualizing achievement.

Step 8: Commit and Take Action (5 minutes)
In your journal, jot down a commitment statement declaring your devotion to these new routines. Take action right away to begin one of the habits after that. Setting up a reminder on your phone or taking the first baby step toward your habit goal could suffice.
Step 9: Monitor Your Development (Continued)

Use habit-tracking software or your notebook to track your development every day or once a week. Keep track of your achievements, setbacks, and any changes you make. You can see your development and maintain accountability by tracking your progress.

Step 10: Consider and Make Changes (Continued)

Review your habit designs regularly and consider your experiences. Are your chosen habits still in line with your values and objectives? Do you need to change anything or acquire any new behaviors? Keep the habit-forming process flexible and active.

Connecting this activity with your beliefs and goals can be a meaningful springboard for forming new habits. It aids in your prioritization, habit-defining, and commitment to positive change. Remember that developing habits takes time, and this first action is the start of your road toward transformation.

CHAPTER 4:
MINDFUL MORNINGS AND VALUES

The Impact of Starting the Day Aligned with Values

Starting the day aligned with your values can profoundly and positively impact your overall well-being and sense of purpose. Your values are the core principles and beliefs that guide your actions, decisions, and priorities in life. When you intentionally begin your day by connecting with these values, you set a powerful tone for the hours ahead. Here are some key impacts of starting your day aligned with your values.

When you wake up with a clear understanding of your values, you have a sense of purpose that can sharpen your focus. You know what truly matters to you, and this clarity helps you filter out distractions and prioritize activities aligned with your values. As a result, you can approach your day with a heightened sense of purpose and direction.

Aligning your morning routine with your values can boost your motivation and drive. Your values are a source of intrinsic motivation, providing the "why" behind your actions. When you start your day by engaging in activities that resonate with your values, you're more likely to feel energized and inspired to tackle challenges and enthusiastically pursue your goals.

Life often presents unexpected challenges and stressors. However, when your day begins with a grounding in your values, you're better equipped to face adversity with resilience. Your values are a source of inner strength, helping you stay true to your principles even in difficult circumstances.

Values-based mornings empower you to make decisions that align with your long-term goals and beliefs. When faced with choices throughout the day, you can refer to your core values to guide your decision-making process. This leads to more intentional choices and a greater sense of personal integrity.

Starting the day aligned with your values contributes to greater well-being. Engaging in activities and habits that reflect your values can enhance your emotional and mental health. It fosters a sense of authenticity, self-acceptance, and inner peace, which are essential components of overall well-being.

Your values influence how you interact with others. You'll likely engage in empathetic and compassionate behavior when you begin the day with a values-oriented mindset. This may lead to stronger and more meaningful connections with friends, family, and colleagues, as your actions reflect your commitment to your values.

Aligned with your values, you're more likely to focus on tasks and projects that matter most to you. This heightened focus and motivation can increase productivity and a greater sense of accomplishment as you work toward your goals with purpose and intention.

Ultimately, starting the day aligned with your values contributes to a deeper sense of fulfillment and satisfaction. You're living a life that reflects your authentic self and what you hold dear. This alignment with your values can bring profound and lasting joy and contentment.

Incorporating values-based practices into your morning routine can take various forms, such as journaling, meditation, or setting daily intentions that align with your values. The specific practices you choose should resonate with you personally and remind you what truly matters in your life. Regardless of your methods, starting the day aligned with your values extends beyond the morning hours, influencing the quality and direction of your entire day and, ultimately, your life.

Practical Tips: Establishing a Values-Driven Morning Routine

Creating a morning ritual based on your values can change your life by giving you a sense of direction and focus throughout the day. To help you establish a morning routine that reflects your values, here are some suggestions:

To get started, think about what matters most to you. What do you hold to be the most important values and beliefs? Create a list of the most important things to you and reflect on how they affect your relationships, work, health, and development.

Realize that it's unrealistic to expect your daily routine to accommodate all of your principles. Focus on the principles that mean the most to you right now. By doing so, you may keep your daily activities organized and manageable.

It would be best if you remembered your day's goals before getting out of bed. Choose the exact activities and behaviors you'll take to demonstrate your principles. Defining goals can bring your attitude into harmony with your ideals.

Create time in your morning routine to reflect on your beliefs. It might be anything from a comfy chair to writing in a secluded nook for meditation. Create an atmosphere that encourages thought and self-examination here.

Keeping a journal might help you get in touch with your core beliefs. Get all you can think of about your values down on paper. Use diary prompts that make you think about how you can act in ways that are consistent with your values.

Try starting your day with some quiet time spent meditating or practicing mindfulness. Take a deep breath, think about what matters most, and mentally prepare yourself for the day ahead. Focusing on your ideals during a guided meditation or breathing exercise can have profound effects.

Make sure your values are reflected in your affirmations. If you repeat these to yourself daily, you can strengthen your resolve to act according to your principles. Consider the virtue of "kindness" and the statement, "I choose kindness in all my interactions today."

Take part in a mental exercise in which you imagine yourself living by your ideals. Imagine concrete examples of how living your ideals has a beneficial effect on your life.

Change your morning routine to reflect your principles. For example, if "health" is important to you, try incorporating some form of physical activity, a healthy breakfast, or a mindfulness practice into your morning routine.

Schedule in the mornings some time to focus on your values. Select a time slot, even if it's only 15–30 minutes per day, that you can consistently stick to.

Reality often throws curveballs. It's important to be flexible with your daily schedule. Being adaptable does not imply letting your principles go in favor of a more convenient situation.

Tell someone you trust about your new values-based morning routine so they can help keep you on track. You can find help from people who share your ideals by joining an online community.

Check-in regularly to see if your morning routine is helping you live a life consistent with your values. Adjust as necessary to maintain harmony.

Creating a morning routine based on your principles takes time and effort. Try to be kind to yourself as you make this a regular habit. Even baby steps toward a life more aligned with your ideals are progress worth celebrating.

Using these guidelines, you can create a morning routine that helps you have a productive day and gives you the tools to make decisions that align with your beliefs and goals.

Experiments and Adjustments in Morning Practices

Experimenting with different morning routines is a natural and important component of habit-building and personal development. They allow you to adjust your routine to changing circumstances and match your morning rituals with your values and objectives. Here are some reasons why trying new things and making changes is important, as well as some tips for doing so:

1. Accepting Growth and Change:

Your values, priorities, and circumstances may change since life is dynamic. What was beneficial for you is no longer applicable or useful. Being open to experimenting with new morning routines that more accurately reflect your present goals and values is necessary to embrace change and growth.

2. Discovering What Really Works:

Iteration lets you identify the morning rituals that speak to you the most. By experimenting with various strategies, you can discover the routines and habits that improve your well-being, productivity, and alignment with your values. Discovering your own special recipe for a fulfilling morning is the goal of this procedure.

3. Overcoming Static and Plateaus:

You can occasionally believe your morning routine has reached a ceiling or stopped evolving. This indicates that changes need to be made. You can escape the routine and give your morning routines new vitality through experimentation.

4. Adaptability and Flexibility:

Too much rigidity in your morning routine can make you angry when unplanned circumstances derail your intentions. Trying new things and making changes helps you become more adaptable. You can design a routine that is adaptable enough to handle changes without compromising your beliefs.

5. Addressing Obstacles and Challenges:

In your morning rituals, experimentation is a useful tool for overcoming obstacles. Experimenting with various strategies can help you find answers that work for you if you constantly struggle with a certain component of your routine.

How to Approach Morning Practice Experiments and Modifications
Before altering your morning routine, clearly define the goals or outcomes you hope to attain. Do you want to be more productive, feel better, or be more in line with your values?
Start Small: When testing out new procedures, start with minor adjustments. To prevent overloading yourself, introduce one new behavior or change at a time. This enables you to accurately assess the effects of each adjustment.

Keep a Journal: Keep a journal to record the results of your investigations. Keep track of how each change impacts your mood, level of energy, and general well-being. This notebook can aid in deciding which procedures to preserve and which to tweak further.

Be Consistent: Allow enough time for each experiment's results to be seen. Consistency is essential to determine whether a practice is in line with your beliefs and objectives. A few days of experimentation might not produce any insightful results.

Ask for feedback: Talk to dependable family members, friends, or mentors about your experiments and revisions. They can offer insightful viewpoints and assist you in identifying potential blind spots.

Evaluate and Reflect: Analyze the outcomes of your trials regularly. Consider whether each activity is consistent with your values and whether it adds value to your life. Prepare yourself to get rid of habits that no longer benefit you.

Iterate and Change: Morning routines might change. Be prepared to modify and improve your routine as necessary. Open to new opportunities because what works today might not work in a year.

Experimentation can include trial and error, so be patient and kind to yourself. Be kind to yourself while you adjust to these changes, and try not to be too hard on yourself if some of your experiments don't produce the outcomes you were hoping for.

A great method to ensure that your morning routine stays in line with your beliefs and objectives is to incorporate experiments and changes. It helps you live a more rewarding and purpose-driven existence by keeping your mornings interesting, reflective of your ever-changing objectives, and fresh.

CHAPTER 5: THE WORK-LIFE BALANCE EQUATION

Ensuring Your Work Habits Reflect Your Core Values

Making your work habits consistent with your principles is crucial to experiencing professional satisfaction, honesty, and harmony. Your values are the concepts and beliefs you hold dearest, and you should never put them separately from your professional life. Here are some ways to make sure your work habits are in line with who you really are:

Identifying your fundamental beliefs is the first step. In your professional and personal life, what do you hold to be the most significant principles, ethics, and beliefs? It would be best if you took the time to choose which of these values is most important to you, as they will form the basis for how you conduct yourself at work.

Think about how you normally go about your workday. Do they support or go against who you really are as a person? Time management, decision-making, communication, teamwork, and ethics should all be figured into your evaluation.

Create professional objectives that are in line with who you really are. Your values should inform the details of these objectives. If "integrity" is one of your values, resolve to conduct yourself professionally at all times.

Communicate your values to your coworkers and superiors. Being transparent about your beliefs may help others grasp them and create an environment where they are valued.

Remember your values and use them as a compass when making important decisions at work. Before deciding, consider whether it helps you maintain your personal and professional honor.

Think over what you have to do each day. Examine how you better integrate this work with your personal ideals. If "teamwork" is one of your values, seek ways to work together and encourage your coworkers.

Maintain a good work-life balance by making changes to your daily routine. Maintaining this equilibrium helps you prioritize things like family, health, and self-improvement, all essential to your happiness.

Create firm limits at work to shield your principles and yourself from potential violations. This could mean saying no to assignments that go against your ideals or standing up for yourself in tense situations.

Prioritize opportunities aligning with your values while considering a job or career transition. Do homework on potential employers or roles to see if their culture and beliefs mesh with yours.

Recognize that bringing your work practices into harmony with your ideals is a never-ending task. Adapt to your changing circumstances by welcoming the idea of continual improvement and being amenable to adjusting your routine accordingly.

To better connect your work habits with your principles, seek advice and criticism from mentors, peers, or a coach. They can give you good advice and keep you honest.

Maintain honesty and sincerity in all of your endeavors. Maintain a continuous alignment between your actions and your values. Being genuine earns you the respect and trust of your peers and superiors.

A more satisfying working life can be achieved by deliberately incorporating personal values into daily job activities and major decisions. This harmony improves not just your sense of accomplishment in your work but also the morale and health of everyone around you.

Strategies to Negotiate and Navigate Workplace Challenges

It might be difficult to overcome obstacles in the office, but with the correct approach, you can improve your work life and the lives of others around you. Here are some useful tactics for discussing and solving problems at work:

Effective Communication

The ability to articulate one's thoughts clearly and concisely is foundational to solving problems head-on in the business. Active listening is a crucial part of this process. Active listening entails paying undivided focus to the speaker. This requires listening to them and considering their points of view, emotions, and goals. Active listening is essential to effectively develop answers and foster productive connections in the workplace.

Equally important is speaking one's mind confidently and clearly. If you want your views, worries, and ideas to be heard and respected, you must express them clearly and confidently. However, you must treat each other with dignity at all times. Conflicts can develop when assertiveness is misunderstood as hostility. Instead, it means being open to other people's points of view while being firm in your own.

One of the best ways to improve morale and productivity on the job is to encourage open communication among employees. It's much easier to foster an environment where people trust one another and are willing to work together when they know they may voice their opinions and thoughts without fear of retaliation. When employees are encouraged to share their thoughts and feelings, possible issues can be identified early, and solutions can be discussed rationally. A more peaceful and productive workplace results when conflicts are resolved amicably and misconceptions are minimized.

Conflict Resolution

Employees who can resolve conflicts effectively can substantially facilitate a happy and productive work atmosphere. Maintaining composure and objectivity is a crucial skill in dispute resolution. It's normal for tempers to flare when problems arise. However, letting your emotions control your behavior can make the situation worse. Keeping your cool allows for more level headed debate and decision-making. Understand the problem at hand and deal with it calmly and rationally rather than responding emotionally.

One effective method for resolving conflicts is to find a solution that benefits everyone involved. Seek win-win solutions to problems instead of treating them as zero-sum games in which one side must lose for the other to win. This calls for a cooperative and accommodating frame of mind. It's all about compromising and making things work well for everyone involved. By focusing on mutually beneficial outcomes, you can improve your relationships with coworkers and reduce the likelihood of future confrontations.

Sometimes, it won't go away, no matter how hard you try to resolve a disagreement. When this occurs, it may be wise to bring in a mediator to help sort things out. A mediator is an impartial third party who can help participants in an argument communicate with one another. A mediator might be anyone from a superior to an HR representative to an impartial third party. Mediation is useful for resolving difficult issues because it offers an objective viewpoint. It promotes honest discussion, increasing the likelihood of finding long-term solutions to problems. Using a mediator shows that the company cares about resolving conflicts fairly and wants to keep the peace at work, which is good for everyone.

Adaptability

The degree to which you can adapt to new situations at work is a major factor in how well you do. Being adaptable and open to new ideas is more vital than ever in today's competitive job market. Here is a broader perspective on the value of adaptability:

The ability to adapt to new conditions, whether they involve a change in responsibilities, an upgrade in technology, or a reorganization within the company, is what we mean when we talk about flexibility. You can take things as they come and adapt quickly with a flexible mindset. Your ability to adjust to new circumstances quickly will serve you well in today's fast-paced job. Flexibility makes you a more valuable employee by increasing your ability to take on new responsibilities, integrate into new teams, and deal with the unexpected. This will not only help you succeed in the face of adversity, but it will also establish you as an indispensable asset to your company.

Acceptance of change requires more than just a pliable attitude. Embracing change means viewing each new experience as possible to learn and develop new skills. You embrace change as an opportunity to develop instead of something to be feared. By maintaining a constructive frame of mind, you can use setbacks as opportunities for growth. It allows you to keep your interest and energy in your profession high, which can be contagious to those around you. To effectively contribute to your organization's success, you must adapt to new circumstances.

Maintaining composure in the face of disruption is the definition of adaptability, while actively seeking growth and improvement in any and all workplace changes is the essence of embracing change. These two facets of flexibility operate in tandem to make you capable of handling the workplace's ups and downs with poise and thriving in and making meaningful contributions to an environment that is always shifting and growing.

Emotional Intelligence

Emotional intelligence, or EQ, refers to a collection of abilities that can significantly impact how well you handle stressful situations at work and how well you get along with your coworkers. In this article, we will examine two of the most important aspects of emotional intelligence:

The development of one's own self-awareness is the cornerstone of emotional quotient. Understanding your own feelings, causes, and responses is essential. Being in touch with your emotions allows you to see how they shape your actions and judgments. Being self-aware makes you better control your feelings, which is especially helpful at trying times so that you don't act rashly or make poor decisions.

Another benefit of developing self-awareness is the ability to step back and evaluate one's reactions. Suppose you feel defensive during a work dispute, for instance. In that case, you can take stock of your feelings and consider how you would respond more constructively and rationally if you were more self-aware. You can keep cool and act professionally, even under intense pressure or experiencing strong emotions.

Self-awareness also allows you to pinpoint specific facets of your character that could use tweaking. Suppose you know patterns in your behavior holding you back professionally or personally. In that case, you can take measures to change them. In the end, your self-awareness will positively impact your interactions with coworkers and your resilience in the face of adversities at work, making it a cornerstone of emotional intelligence.

Empathy is being able to put oneself in another person's shoes and feel what they are feeling and experiencing. Empathizing with others is crucial for success in interpersonal interactions and dispute resolution on the job. Empathy is the mental state in which one actively seeks to understand another person's thoughts, feelings, and experiences, such as a coworker.

Empathy can be an effective strategy for preventing disagreements from escalating when used under trying circumstances. Empathizing with people and acknowledging their feelings is a cornerstone of building trusting relationships. This can facilitate more honest and fruitful conversations, leading to improved problem-solving and conflict resolution.

The ability to empathize also improves your working interactions with other people. People are more open to working together when they believe their contributions will be valued. Leaders and teammates who exhibit empathy are likelier to be liked and trusted by their subordinates and coworkers.

In conclusion, recognizing and understanding your own emotions and those of others is a crucial part of having high levels of emotional intelligence. Empathy aids you connect with others on a deeper level, while self-awareness helps you control your emotions and behaviors, which are useful in the workplace for better communication, dispute resolution, and creating relationships.

Problem-Solving Skills

Effective problem-solving abilities equip you to take on problems and make educated judgments in the business, making them useful. Let's talk about the importance of critical thinking and the development of original approaches to problems.

Critical Thinking

Critical thinking is analyzing, evaluating, and synthesizing information to generate well-informed opinions and choices. To do this, one must consider the topic from multiple angles and weigh the consequences and results. Critical thinking in the workplace enables you to

Evaluate Complicated Matters: Critical thinking helps you dissect a difficult problem into more manageable chunks. The major concerns can be isolated, pertinent data collected, and the relative importance of each element assessed.

Make Informed Decisions: When you employ critical thinking skills, decisions can be made with more forethought and consideration. You think about the here-and-now and far-off future, and you make decisions consistent with who you want to be and what you value.

Identify Assumptions and Biases: The process of critical thinking forces you to become aware of and evaluate your own preconceived notions and biases. It motivates you to look for contrasting arguments and avoid making hasty judgments.

Solve Problems Efficiently: Efficient Problem-Solving Strategies and Methods Can Be Created Through the Application of Critical Thinking. You're more inclined to go to the bottom of things and fix them instead of wasting time on band-aids.

Alternative Methods

To solve problems creatively, one must be able to think in novel ways and try different tactics. It promotes the development of novel ideas and the identification of previously unrecognized approaches to problems. Creative problem-solving at work can:

Take on Complicated Problems: Not all problems at work can be solved with a simple answer. Thinking creatively about problems and developing novel solutions is essential in today's fast-paced world.

Promote Collaboration: Encourage group efforts to solve problems and generate new ideas by holding brainstorming sessions. Each team member brings something special to the table, which can help the group develop better, more comprehensive solutions.

Adapt to Change: To keep up with the ever-changing demands of today's businesses and consumers, it's important to think on your feet and develop innovative solutions to problems. It encourages creative problem-solving and quick thinking.

Improve Your Ability to Make Choices: Coming up with original answers frequently requires considering and settling on one of several novel approaches. Decisions made using this method are more likely to be well-considered and consistent with the company's principles.

Workplace problems can be daunting, but you'll be better prepared to handle them if you include critical thinking and creative problem-solving into your routine. These abilities not only aid in overcoming challenges but also help you develop as a person and in your career, making you an asset in any field.

Time Management

Effective time management is a pillar for handling professional challenges and maintaining productivity. Setting priorities and making good plans are two important parts of time management:

Prioritization

Putting activities and responsibilities in order of importance and urgency entails prioritizing them. It involves making thoughtful choices about how to spend your time and energy. Prioritization is beneficial in the workplace in several ways:

Reducing Stress: By prioritizing your tasks, you may first deal with the top priorities, lessening the stress frequently associated with approaching deadlines or significant deliverables.

Productivity: Setting priorities helps you make the most of your time. You significantly advance toward your goals by completing high-impact tasks first.

Alignment with Goals: Prioritization ensures that you are working on things that align with your goals and values, boosting your sense of accomplishment and purpose.

Time management: You can manage your workload effectively by allocating your time to the most important things. By doing this, time lost on less important tasks is avoided.
The Eisenhower Matrix, which divides jobs into four quadrants depending on urgency and importance, is one method for prioritizing work. You can proactively handle job issues and keep control of your workload by continuously identifying and taking care of things in the "important and urgent" quadrant.

Successful Planning

Making timetables, to-do lists, and techniques to keep you organized and on track is the process of effective planning. It involves managing your time well to have the resources and concentration required to finish activities effectively. In the workplace, excellent planning has the following benefits:

Organization: By making timetables and to-do lists, you can keep track of your chores and make sure that no vital duties fall through the gaps.

Time Allocation: Good planning lets you set aside particular time blocks for various tasks. For tasks requiring intense focus, you could schedule uninterrupted time.

Goal achievement: Planning enables you to divide larger tasks or objectives into more manageable chunks. This makes it simpler to monitor development and accomplish long-term goals.

Reduced Procrastination: You are less likely to put off doing something or waste time on it when you have a clear plan. Your day's work is guided by your plan.

Use time management tools such as calendars, task management apps, or paper planners to efficiently arrange your weekdays. You can use these tools to visualize your timetable, establish due dates, and monitor your progress. You may manage your time better and overcome professional challenges more successfully if you constantly prioritize tasks and plan well. This will also help you strike a healthy work-life balance.

Achieving Balance: Maintaining Boundaries and Sanity

Maintaining your mental health and general contentment requires balancing your personal and professional lives. Maintaining boundaries and keeping your sanity in the chaos of contemporary work environments depend heavily on this balance. Let's look at ways to attain this balance:

Putting Boundaries in Place

A crucial first step in finding balance is establishing clear boundaries between your personal and professional lives. Here is how to go about it:

Define Working Hours: Establish particular working hours to the demands of your position. Avoid the temptation to overwork by adhering as closely as possible to these hours.

Establish a Separate Workstation: Even if you work from home, set up a workstation separate from your living area. This facilitates the mental separation of work and play.

Use Tech Mindfully: Use technology wisely and be aware of how it affects your boundaries. Establish limits for checking work-related emails and texts after hours to avoid constant connectivity.

Share Your Boundaries: Be sure to share your boundaries with family, friends, and coworkers. They should know your availability for work-related matters and your demand for uninterrupted personal time.

Making Self-Care a Priority

Maintaining your sanity and finding equilibrium requires practicing self-care. How to prioritize self-care is as follows:

Set Aside Personal Time: Schedule time for leisurely pursuits, such as exercising, spending time with loved ones, or engaging in a favorite pastime.

Practice awareness: To reduce stress and stay present, incorporate mindfulness techniques, like deep breathing exercises or meditation, into your everyday routine.

Get Enough Sleep: Make sleep a priority by creating a regular sleep routine and relaxing environment. For both physical and emotional health, getting good sleep is essential.

Keep Healthy Habits: Eat balanced meals, drink plenty of water, and exercise frequently. A sound body helps a sound mind.

Practice Saying No

An effective technique for setting limits and establishing balance is saying no. Here's an efficient way to go about it:

Assess Your Present Commitments: Consider your present obligations in both your professional and personal lives. Saying no or renegotiating your involvement is an option if something doesn't fit your priorities or is too much.

Communicate tactfully: Be respectful and explicit when denying a request or promise. Give your justifications and some alternatives.

Seek Assistance

If you struggle to maintain balance or deal with overwhelming issues, don't be afraid to ask for help from mentors, coworkers, friends, or mental health experts. Speaking with a person who can relate to your situation can be a great way to get advice and emotional support.

Finally, finding balance while upholding your limits and retaining your sanity is a continuous effort that calls for self-awareness, attentive time management, and good communication. You may lead a happier and more balanced life, both personally and professionally, by establishing clear boundaries, placing self-care first, prioritizing it, using your time wisely, learning to say no when required, and getting support when required.

CHAPTER 6:
VALUE-CENTERED RELATIONSHIPS AND COMMUNICATION.

Building Relationships with Communication and Respect

Imagine hanging out with your best friend and being completely at ease while you two almost read each other's minds. It's strange but interesting. This kind of close relationship doesn't happen by accident. It's constructed piece by piece on a solid foundation of respect and communication. If you've ever wondered, "Man, how do I get more of that goodness in my life?" you're lucky because cultivating and honing the talent of creating connections with these two essential components isn't some mysterious art. So, if you're up for the adventure, pull up a soft chair and join us as we explore the warm world of intelligent communication and sincere respect.

Imagine there are countless delicious, complicated, and perhaps baffling relationship recipes. Like different components in a cuisine, each conversation, moment of stillness, and nuanced expression of affection contribute to the extraordinary complexity of your connection.

Consider the following: You, the relationship chef, are responsible for transforming individual ingredients into a savory whole through the effective and creative use of various communication strategies. And remember, friend, that effective communication requires the same careful, delicate balancing of different parts as good cuisine. One of the most important factors? Indeed, this is a form of active listening.

Envision yourself carrying a bowl full of your loved one's most tender feelings and thoughts. My buddy, active listening is like holding that bowl in your hands and cradling it with all your concentration so that you can smell the delicate nuances of the underlying emotions and hear the wordless echoes of the unspoken feelings and intents beneath the surface.

You're doing more than just listening when you open your mind, eyes, and heart to what's being said and unsaid around you. When you show the person you're talking to that you understand them and care about what they say, it's as if you give them a big, comforting embrace. It's like taking your time to slowly simmer a sauce so that the tastes may really come together while still honoring the individual qualities of each component.

There's even more to the recipe than that! Consider the part that patience plays in how you cook up your messages. Allowing the other person to finish their thoughts before jumping to conclusions, like a stew that has been allowed to slowly cook to bring out all of its flavors. It's about allowing the emotions, ideas, and words to slowly stew, developing into a profound and genuine conversation.

In addition, let's season your meal with empathy, a vital ingredient in effective communication. It's a fine art that requires putting oneself in one position, seeing the world as one does, feeling what one feels, and experiencing what they have. The secret to a successful blend is a slow, steady swirl incorporating all ingredients without overworking the mixture.

Oh, and now I see! Think of it as the perfect seasoning for your message. When you communicate your thoughts, feelings, and intentions clearly, the receiver will perceive them as you intended: clearly, distinctly, and truthfully. Your message should be as distinct and enjoyable as the individual components of a well-prepared meal.

What do you get when you put active listening together with patience, empathy, and clarity in the communication kitchen? A connection like the one you're creating is like a heartfelt feast that nourishes, fulfills, and magnificently enriches both parties.

Imagine having the most wonderful conversation in which you express your emotions while the person next to you is looking at their phone. It's a little depressing. Respect in conversation is equivalent to treating the person in front of you like a VIP. No matter how dissimilar, their opinions are respected and taken into account. It's about giving people room to speak without interruption, nodding in agreement, and responding in a way that communicates, "I see you, I hear you, and you matter."

Real encounters between people are the building blocks of strong relationships, and mutual respect is the landscaping. Every conversation nourishes the seeds of connection, allowing them to grow into the magnificent tree of companionship and trust. It's a journey, not a sprint. And what's this? You have what it takes, my friend, to excel at developing relationships and creating solid and heartwarming links in their breadth and authenticity.

Habitual Kindness, Listening, and Respectful Discourse

Kindness

However great they are, occasional acts of kindness and benevolence at random are not what we mean when we talk of continuous compassion. Instead, visualize persistent kindness as a mellow, understated tune that lulls you to sleep with every encounter and becomes integral to who you are. It happens when your compassion is a continual presence, bringing a lovely, kind tone to your actions, words, and gestures.

Imagine sending a message to someone, possibly something little and insignificant at first glance, but enveloping it in the warmth that makes them feel seen, cared for, and important. It's similar to offering a virtual embrace that is cushioned by words that have been carefully and thoughtfully chosen. Your thoughtful comments become a beacon of empathy and connection in a time when internet exchanges frequently lack the warmth of a personal presence, navigating the vast digital space to subtly touch a soul.

Let's apply that idea to our encounters in the real world. Imagine entering a room and radiating genuine joy at each person's presence rather than just saying "hello" as you enter. It's your eyes shining as you meet theirs, a genuine smile that spreads with ease, and words that are infused with genuine interest and care despite speaking about commonplace subjects. Your generosity creates a reassuring, calming influence that encourages honesty and faith.

And oh, the enchantment it weaves in hard times! When approached with kindness, encountering disagreements and conflicts— unavoidable companions of human interactions—becomes a totally different experience. Imagine negotiating a difficult conversation when your words are restrained by empathy and understanding, even when expressing disagreement or disappointment. It involves speaking your truth without casting a shadow over another person's viewpoint. Then, your compassion goes beyond simply soothing; it also strengthens the area by creating a sense of safety that promotes openness and vulnerability.

Consider the connections you make when kindness is a regular feature of your interactions rather than a passing visitor. It transforms into a soft link that binds souls, a quiet reassurance that "you're in a safe place," and a strong connection that endures even when the bonds of understanding fall apart. Your consistent kindness creates a song that stays in relationships, whether long-lasting friendships, romantic partnerships, or casual encounters. This melody is frequently the solace that people seek out and treasure.

Imagine the haven your routine kindness offers in a society that frequently hums with hurried exchanges and fleeting encounters. Being a real, ongoing source of warmth, compassion, and caring is more important than simply being pleasant. The goal is to develop into a person whose very existence becomes equated with a comforting embrace that softly mutters, "Here you are valued, here you are cared for."

Oh, the intricate web of relationships you create with this supreme, unassuming power of routine kindness is uplifting and soul-stirring in its richness and sincerity. Embracing kindness in this way, making it an integral, seamless part of every conversation, you're not just developing relationships; you're crafting soulful connections that vibrate with the quiet, reassuring hum of true care and understanding.

Listening

The act of listening encompasses more than just hearing. It's an immersive experience that appeals to all the senses, not just hearing but also seeing, thinking, and, most importantly, feeling. It's the atmosphere where your whole being can relax and listen to the harmonious interplay of words, feelings, and the spaces between. Being present with another person and truly listening to them creates an environment where barriers dissolve, masks drop, and hearts open.

Let your mind wander to a time when you were sitting across from a close friend, and they were telling you about their day. It sounds like normal conversation on the surface, but there's a subtle pull on their words that makes you want to dig a little further. When a certain subject arises, they look away or pause for a second before continuing. Here, your intuitive, empathic heart is as important as your ears in picking up on the silent waves of unspoken emotions and thoughts.

Envision your attentiveness as a warm embrace, holding their words and quiet with the same care. Empathetic quiet gently covers the dialogue as judgment gives way to understanding, and counsel takes a back seat. Your thoughtful silence often conveys more than words can, gently saying, "I'm here, you're heard, and it's safe for you to be utterly, beautifully you."

Vulnerabilities are not revealed but shared in this safe place of deep listening, like delicate secrets told between close friends. It's a place where feelings that can't be put into words can be acknowledged and comforted. One person speaks while the other listens, taking in not only the words but also the plethora of feelings, thoughts, and wordless screams between them.

Just think of the relationships established in this safe space of attentiveness. It's the place where acquaintances become friends, and friends create soulful ties that go beyond just words. Where mutual understanding slowly develops, enveloping both parties in a feeling of safety and trust is where true friendship thrives.

What a difference attentive listening makes! To become a confidant is to become a safe space where hearts can unload their deepest worries and discover not solutions but understanding and relief. When your being becomes a serene sea that softly cradles the outpouring of another soul, you become more than just a listener. It's a type of generosity and a silent, powerful one that often forges the loveliest, longest-lasting bonds.

The promise of genuine listening is unspoken, my buddy. A guarantee that says, "Just be yourself around me. There is always room for your thoughts, stillness, and the space in between. Through attentive, empathic listening, relationships may weather the storms of miscommunication and strife, emerging stronger and more connected than before.

Discovering this beautiful art form must be a joy. Just give me the signal, and I'll be more than happy to return to your mind to explore even more dimensions or possibly a whole new topic!

Mitigating Conflicts through Value-Led Dialogues

Imagine a space where different points of view are seen as assets rather than liabilities, allowing everyone in it to learn from one another and grow as a unit. Having a conversation where values—our most fundamental beliefs and guiding principles—take center stage, especially in tense situations, is a unique and powerful experience.

When problems occur in people's relationships, as they inevitably will, it's not often the major arguments on the surface that cause tension. Despite outward disagreements, our minds and hearts are guided by shared principles that lay under the surface. The seed of compromise can take root only when these ideals are acknowledged, comprehended, and upheld, even amid conflict.

How refreshing it would be if, in conversations, we dueled not with the defensive shields of 'right' and 'wrong' but with the 'whys' that cradle our ideas, digging deeper and learning from one another. Like slowly peeling an onion, it reveals not just the surface differences but also the underlying values, anxieties, and hopes.

By shifting the focus of the discourse to these underlying ideals, it can be transformed from a battleground of competing opinions into a fruitful environment for the growth of mutual understanding and respect. Conflicts are not settled by silencing or eradicating opposing viewpoints but rather by incorporating them into a cohesive whole.

How wonderfully illuminating can conversations centered on shared values be! The dynamic changed when we stopped trying to convince the other person of our point of view and started trying to learn about theirs. No longer is victory in an argument more important than creating a shared environment where different values can exist, sometimes in peaceful concord and other times in respectful tension.

These conversations, especially with high tensions, are like turning on a light in a room with many miscommunications and misconceptions. Softly, it shines a light on the values and beliefs that are often the unseen drivers of our opinions and the obvious, glaring disputes.

Resolution takes on new significance in this comfortably illuminated room. Finding a compromise that placates competing perspectives isn't the goal; it's more important to chart a course that does justice to the ideals at stake. The path to resolution is not always going to be straight and smooth but rather a meandering and sympathetic one that considers and respects the unique set of values that each person brings to the table.

By using dialogues guided by shared values, we can avoid or resolve disputes while shaping a partnership in which our differences are valued and our similarities are recognized. It's about finding common ground in the rich, varied tapestry of values and building bridges across differences.

CONCLUSION

An infinite pool of wisdom can be mined if one sets out on a voyage of introspection through the lens of good practices. Imagine you are on a journey where each footfall is accompanied by the deliberate decision to adopt practices that feed your body, mind, heart, and soul.

Picture yourself developing an attitude of gratitude, wherein you take time off from the ups and downs of life to bask in the glow of appreciation. It's like sprinkling sunshine on bright and dark days, seeing the value and lessons hidden in every circumstance. Imagine the times when you felt an overwhelming sense of gratitude for something, whether it was the laughter of a loved one, the embrace of your bed after a long day, or the soft whisper of the breeze on your face. It's a practice that subtly weaves moments of joy and hope into the otherwise monotonous fabric of existence.

Now, gradually incorporate the practice of being in the here and now into your travels. Envision yourself participating in the events around you rather than simply observing them. Allowing yourself to be totally present is like letting go of the past and future so that your thoughts can float effortlessly with the rhythm of the present. Being totally present, soaking in and reflecting the depth and beauty of each moment, makes everything from a friend's laughter to the soothing sound of rain to the mesmerizing dance of a falling leaf immeasurably more lovely.

Let's take a little more time to wander around the habit of kindness, where your words, deeds, and even thoughts are all wrapped up in a warm, loving embrace. Imagine a world where communication is more like art than a simple trade and where kindness, compassion, and love are freely given and received. It's as if you transformed into a calm, comforting tune that warmed the hearts of those around you and nudged them ever so little toward hope and joy. It's a practice that helps you see clearly and acts as a gentle beacon for those around you.

Think about how often you learn new things and how curious you are. Envision your travels being tinged with vivid hues of curiosity, where each encounter, each interaction, and each moment is a goldmine of knowledge and discovery. It's like being on a never-ending journey, one in which every day opens up a new chapter of personal development, new perspectives, and exciting discoveries.

When viewed through the prism of good habits, one's life is like a work of art, where each brushstroke, color, and detail is filled with deliberate, thoughtful decisions that have served to revitalize, elevate, and wonderfully light one's journey. It's not simply a route but a brilliant, vibrant tapestry commemorating the exquisite, profound beauty of life in its whole, as the echoes of love, generosity, gratitude, presence, and eternal learning echo with each footfall.

What a glorious adventure you are setting out on, you lovely individuals, traveling into the domain of healthy routines.

Developing routines that enrich your whole being is more than a trip; it's an exhilarating dance with the universe. It's a journey in which every action and decision you make composes the soundtrack to your life, filling you with a sense of well-being, happiness, and a weightlessness of spirit.

Think of it this way: with every good practice you adopt, you aren't just altering your days and weeks; you're also gently sculpting your very essence, creating pathways that lead to a life that not only pulses with vitality but also radiates an exquisite, subtle joy that springs from your very core. It's about crafting an existence in which health and happiness are not goals to be achieved but byproducts of how you live your life.

Take comfort in knowing that you are not alone in your quest to adopt healthier routines. It's a beautiful dance where everyone participates, and everyone's efforts, successes, and failures are treasured and acknowledged. Every little victory is celebrated as a giant leap toward community health and happiness, and every adversity is met with understanding and compassion.

Remember, lovely spirit, that developing healthy routines is not a predetermined course of action but a graceful dance in which you will find yourself both leading and being led. Your life is a dance, and as you go through it, you'll experience highs and lows, but you'll also gain crucial insights and a complete picture of who you really are due to the lows.

Imagine your journey not as an attempt to achieve perfection but as a warm embrace of the wonderfully flawed person you already are, where each baby step toward healthy routines is a triumphant acknowledgment of your strength, determination, and resolve to fill your life with the soothing light of wellness.

Oh, the people you'll meet, the cultures you'll encounter, the new frontiers you'll learn about, and the possibilities you'll discover on your travels! All the little things you do daily that promote your health and happiness add up to a life that is not merely lived but celebrated, cherished, and infinitely loved.

I pray that your life's path of good choices is like a twirling dance through the rainbow of life's colors, creating moments that you see, feel, absorb, and treasure in the inner sanctuary of your soul.

Here I am, always prepared to walk by you on the enchanted roads of health, exploration, and deep, unbounded joy, should you ever need a few words of encouragement, a little nudge of motivation, or simply a partner to share a moment on this lovely journey.

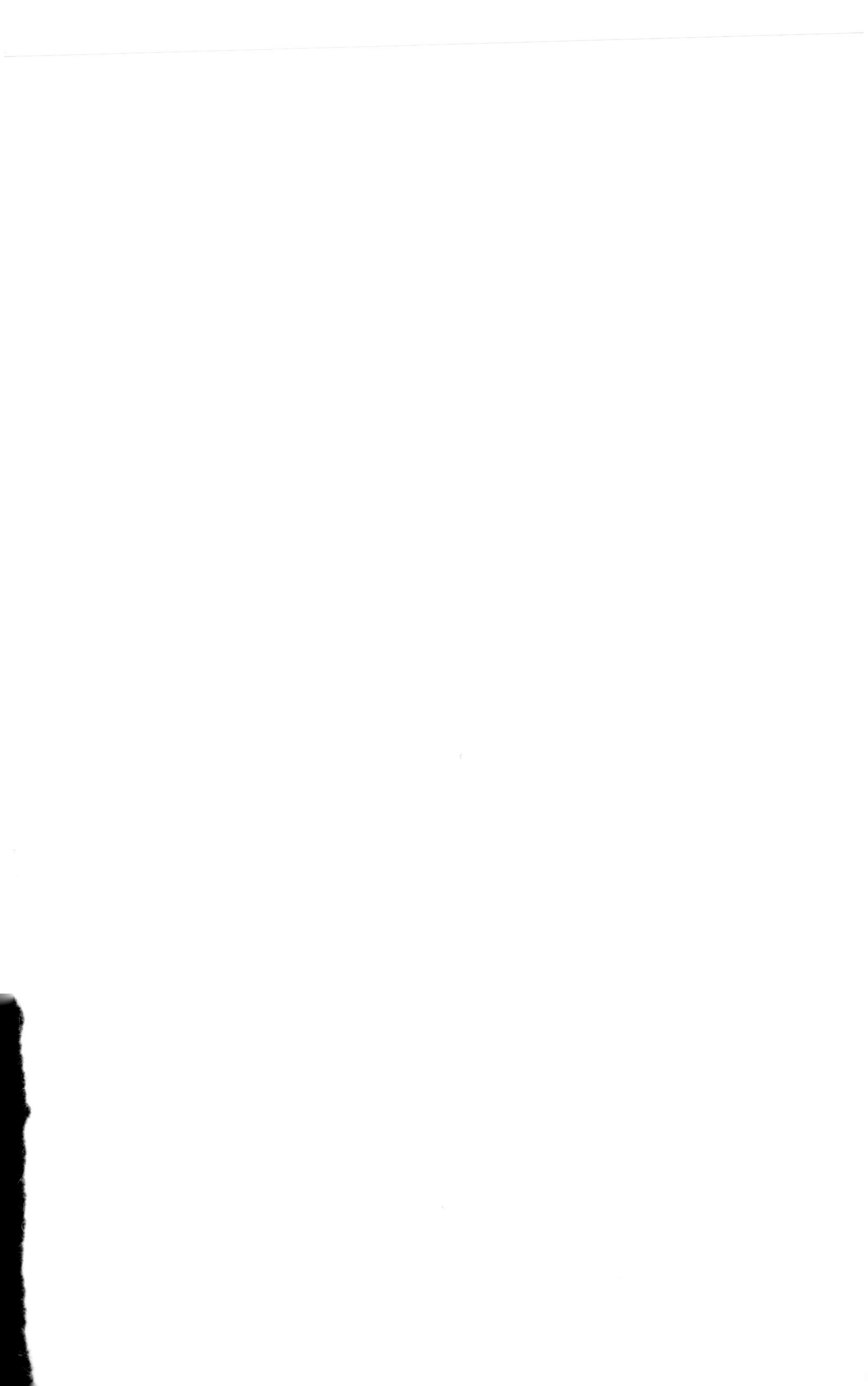

www.ingramcontent.com/pod-product-compliance
Ingram Content Group UK Ltd.
Pitfield, Milton Keynes, MK11 3LW, UK
UKHW062312290726
14090UKWH00018B/1016